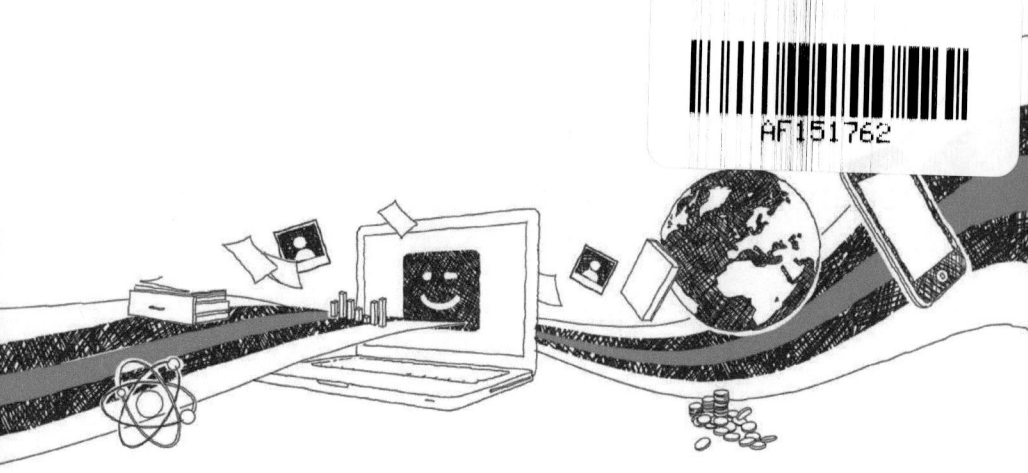

Eye Dominance in Tennis Serve

The Association of Manually Influenced Eye Dominance with the Shoulder Loading Position in a Tennis Serve

Hakan Dahlbo
Michael Flatz

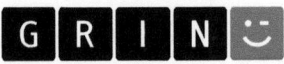

Bibliographic information published by the German National Library:

The German National Library lists this publication in the National Bibliography; detailed bibliographic data are available on the Internet at http://dnb.dnb.de.

ISBN: 9783346696304
This book is also available as an ebook.

© GRIN Publishing GmbH
Nymphenburger Straße 86
80636 München

Print and binding: Books on Demand GmbH, Norderstedt, Germany
Printed on acid-free paper from responsible sources.

The present work has been carefully prepared. Nevertheless, authors and publishers do not incur liability for the correctness of information, notes, links and advice as well as any printing errors.

GRIN web shop: https://www.grin.com/document/1254540

PUBLICATION

Hakan Dahlbo[1], Michael Flatz[2]

[1] University of Nicaragua – Innsbruck, Austria
[2] Department for Sport Science, University of Innsbruck, Austria

Eye dominance in tennis serve: An exploration of shoulder loading position in the tennis serve and its association with manually influenced eye dominance

Corresponding author:

Hakan Dahlbo

University of Central Nicaragua –Innsbruck, Austria

Key words (15)

Ocular dominance, hand-eye coordination, hand-eye interactivity, shoulder position, tennis serve,

Abstract

Manually influenced eye dominance (MIED) seems to be important to analyse the shoulder loading position (SLOP) in the tennis serve. Thirty-one right-handed healthy tennis players underwent SLOP evaluation recorded with an eight-camera VICON system. The current study (Study II=SII) evaluated open and closed SLOPs in comparison with previous presented results on crossed and consistent MIEDs (Study I=SI). The SLOPs were defined as closed ($\geq 90°$) or open ($<90°$) in relation to the baseline. Firstly, the most common SLOP, closed or open was evaluated. Secondly, whether the most common SLOP is encountered more frequently with crossed respectively consistent MIED classification. The results of SI were compared with the SLOP results of SII. Two eye dominance (ED) tests were compared; Porta Test (PT/P-MIED) and Circular Test (CT/C-MIED). The current study revealed that the closed SLOP was the most common (n=22; p=0.02). The comparative analyses of a stratified sample of SLOP (n=22) with the P-MIED respectively with the C-MIED revealed that 10 out of the 22 closed SLOP players showed crossed P-MIED whereas in the same sample 16 out of the 22 players showed a crossed C-MIED. The analyse of the SLOP/P-MIED is aligned with the results of previous ED studies (p=0.375) whereas the SLOP/C-MIED analyse shows a significant different result (p=0.010) compared to SLOP/P-MIED. The chi-squared test was used to compare the groups. The experiments describe that MIEDs may be efficient to analyse a player's choice of SLOP in the tennis serve. The results may have an impact on serving technique.

Table of Contents

Background

The serve motion seems to show personal variations and individual diversity. Instantly before striking the ball, the player seems to choose a personal shouldersh loading position (SLOP). The kinetic chain is responsible for the energetic flow and is interlinking the energy transport from the legs, throughout the spine to the shoulder (Kovacs & Ellenbecker, 2011). In fact, the production of ground reaction forces is essential for the development of an effective serve (Kibler, 1995; Girard et al., 2005; Elliott et al., 1995). More than 50% of the force and kinetic energy delivered to the shoulder and ultimately to the hand is built up through the legs and trunk work (Kibler, 1995; Toyoshima et al., 1974). The sequence of motions throughout the entire body starts at the lower limbs, through the trunk rotation that leads to upper limb rotation (Elliott et al. 2003). However, if the kinetic chain cannot work fluently without interruption it may limit the performance and enhance the risk of injury. The biomechanic of the serve is commonly divided in 3 phases: 1) preparation phase, 2) acceleration phase, and 3) follow-through phase (Kovacs & Ellenbecker, 2011). During the preparation phase of the serve necessary energy is stored to support the release during the acceleration phase of the stroke (Kovacs & Ellenbecker, 2011). This study is investigating the SLOP as a part of the preparation phase. The SLOP was considered in order to obtain good reliability in the measurement of the current serve study. Certain traits like the personal hand-eye coordination (HEC) preference supposingly may play a role for an impeccable serve motion, however, the gap of knowledge about the SLOPs and the association with manually influenced eye dominance (MIED) is evident. Studies have reported that eye dominance (ED) can shift depending on target direction, but that it cannot shift when in a frontal gaze direction (Khan & Crawford, 2001). However, recent research could show that a circular manually influenced eye dominance (C-MIED) can influence eye dominance switch in a frontal gaze direction (Dahlbo et al. 2020; Study I). Little is known regarding the influence of the HEC patterns in the tennis serve. However, to the best of our knowledge, to date no studies investigated i.e. one-handed motor tasks, similar to the manual grip of a tennis racket, and its specific influence on the ED. In fact, personal hand-eye traits have not devoted any specific attention to the serve development in tennis at all. This study intended to be a first step in that direction. The aim of the study is to explore the MIEDs association with the SLOP in the tennis serve. In particular, the study tests the hypothesis that it is possible to

1

identify an association between the choices of a personal SLOP in the tennis serve with a C-MIED. Indeed, the focus will be on the C-MIED because of its similarity with the manual grip of the tennis racket (Figure 1).

Methods and materials

In order to address critical gaps in the existant literature the study investigated the sample on the most common SLOP in the tennis serve and analysed the association between a personal SLOP and the one-right-handed P-MIED and C-MIED. First, the experiment, evaluated if closed ($\geq 90°$) or open ($<90°$) SLOP in relation to the baseline was more common than was an open loading posititon (Figures 2a and 2b; Table 1); then, the most common SLOP result was compared with P-MIED (A1; Table 2a), Finally, the result of the A1 was compared with the C-MIED results (A2; Table 2b). The Vicon experiment was performed with the same group of players as in SI on MIEDs (Dahlbo et al., 2020). This was necessary in order to compare the SLOP with the P-MIED respectively the C-MIED results. All players in the sample were trained competitive tennis players coached by a qualified certified coach for more than six years. The players were Austrian, German, Italian, Romanian, Russian and Swedish citizens.

The complete study exclusively investigated right-handers. Data were collected from a total of 31 healthy players, nine females (mean ± SD: age 18 ± 4 years, height 171 ± 4 cm, weight 59 ± 5 kg) and 22 males (mean ± SD: age 23 ± 10 years, height 178 ± 10 cm, weight 70 ± 14 kg), who were free of any medical problems. This convenience sample size of 31 subjects was chosen because there were no preliminary data available to formally calculate sample size. Before commencement of the experiment, the participants were fully informed about the procedures and provided written informed consent. The participants had no previous experience with Vicon testing. The tests were performed at the Department for Sport Science, University of Innsbruck, Austria. The experiment was approved by the Board of Ethical Questions in Science of the University of Innsbruck (Certificate 10/2018), Innsbruck, Austria. Detailed information on background, purpose, study procedure, data and data processing for the experiment in the current study was given to all potential participants before they entered the trials. They were informed vocally that participation was voluntary and that they were free to leave the study at any time. Potential risks of participating in the studies were likely to be small, but minor

2

injuries could not completely be excluded. All data were cleaned and anonymised before any data analysis was performed. The raw data were never transmitted electronically. The data is stored at the University of Innsbruck.

Procedure performance

The results of SI (Dahlbo et al., 2020) were used to compare the results with the current study (SII); A circular manual motor Task (CT) with the thumb and the index finger, similar to the grip of a tennis racket (Figure 1), seems to influence the ED.

Figure 1: *Circular grip of the racket*

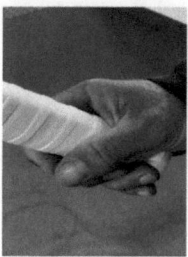

Description of the CT performance (SI)

"The CT Test is a procedure for investigating the manual influence of the eye through a specific circular finger motion (Figure 2b; SI). The subject forms a circle (a hole, Figure 2b; SI) with the index finger and the thumb of the right hand and holds it in front of both wide-open eyes. The right arm is bent approximately 45 degrees. With both eyes open the subject looks through the circle at a specific target (at least five meters away). When instructed, the right eye is closed and if the target can still be seen with the left eye through the finger circle a crossed C-MIED is indicated (right hand/left eye). A consistent C-MIED is given when a right hand/right eye is detected" (Dahlbo et al., 2020).

3

Experiment SLOP in the tennis serve

The biomechanical serve study is based on the 8-stage model by Kovacs and Ellenbecker for tennis serve analysis and focuses on the loading stage of the preparation phase. Specifically, the study investigated closed and open SLOP frequency:

"The components usually seen in the traditional throwing analysis 30, 35 have been altered in this proposed 8-stage tennis-specific serve model. The 8-stage model has 3 distinct phases: preparation, acceleration, and follow-through. Each stage is a direct result of muscle activation and technical adjustments made in the previous stage. When a serve is evaluated, the total body perspective is just as important as the individual segments alone" (Kovacs & Ellenbecker, 2011).

Three-dimensional (3D) analysis is considered to be the gold standard in movement analysis (Ford et al., 2007) and the most recognized and prefered method when researchers are investigating the biomechanic of the serve. The use of 3D motion analysis made it it possible for researchers to investigate the biomechanical and kinetic demands on upper limb loads that contribute to upper extremity injury in tennis serve (Martin et al., 2013; Elliott et al., 2003; Girard et al., 2007; Martin et al. 2014; Elliott & Wood, 1983; Campbell et al., 2013). The 8-stage descriptive model of normal serve mechanics derived from the 3D literature and provided readers with a detailed breakdown of proper mechanics (Kovacs & Ellenbecker, 2011). It described specific body positions and motions and presented the accompanying joint forces and rotational velocities during all the different phases of motion (Kovacs & Ellenbecker, 2011).

Data analysis

To analyse the current study on whether the **closed** SLOP or the **open** SLOP is the most common (Figures 2a and 2b) chi-squared calculation with one-sample test was used. The observed values were compared with the expected values. For the comparing SLOPs/MIEDs analysis (A1 and A2) stratified sampling (n=22) was included (to ensure an adequate subgroup) to compare the frequency of the most common SLOP, closed or open, with the most common one-handed P-MIED respectiviely C-MIED group, crossed or consistent (Figure 6; Table 2a and 2b). Due to the fact that no studies have shown that

4

players choose different positions in the SLOP the values expected for the experiment were equally distributed (50% closed SLOP and 50% open SLOP; Table 1).

In situ capture.

The experiment took place in an indoor laboratory at the Department for Sport Science, University of Innsbruck, Austria. The Vicon tests were performed in a standardized setting with 8 cameras. The SLOP (shoulder orientation line in relation to the baseline; Figure 2a, 2b, 4 and 5) was recorded with eight cameras (Vicon Bonita 10, 200 Hz). The SLOP in the serve was defined as a „closed" position ($\geq 90°$; more clockwise towards 1pm) or an „open" position ($<90°$; more clockwise towards 11am) in relation to the baseline. The players wore their own shoes and sports underwear. All players used the same racket (Head Radical MP™). Thirty-one digitalized standard body location landmarks, 4 markers at the head band and 2 markers on the 2 wrists, 5 racket landmarks, 2 baseline landmarks and soft tennis balls approved by the International Tennis Federation (ITF) were used in a standard setting (Figures 3, 4 and 5).

Protocol

A virtual baseline was prepared on the floor five meters away from the target. Sport tape (white) was used to indicate the baseline (Figure 4 and 5). After warming up (personal program as in usual training program, at least fifteen minutes), each athlete took twenty imaginary swings (serve movements) without a ball in order to familiarize himself with the test equipment. These movements included set-up, loading, cocking/jumping and ending. Each athlete also took some swings with a ball to adjust to the soft ball. Each measurement followed a certain routine. The subject had to execute calibration preparation movements to avoid recording errors. Recording took place before and during the full swing and at ball impact. Biomechanical analysis concentrated on the shoulder position in relation to the baseline during the loading position (Figures 2a, 2b, 4 and 5). The players were told to hit the ball as hard as possible (the way they always hit) into a protected plywood wall with a red target circle (0.5 x 0.5 m) approximately five (5) meters away from the test lab baseline (Figure 4).

Each athlete performed ten serves. Recording errors by some players (marker loss or inability to detect markers during the labeling process) meant that only the first five

5

measurable (out of ten) recorded trials could be chosen as parameter value. Consequently, the mean of the SLOP was calculated from each player's first five recorded trials.

Figure 2a

Closed (5a.i and iv) open (5a.ii and 2b) and shoulder-loading positions (SLOP)

i. Closed SLOP   ii. Open SLOP   iii. Axis of SLOP   iv. Closed SLOP

Acromion (marker)

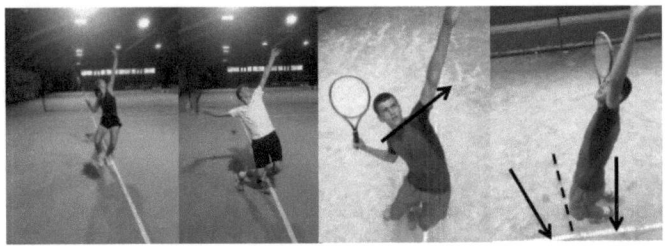

Figure 2b

Shoulder orientation lines description loading position

Baseline: line indicating the boundary of the area of play. (See: In Situ Capture)

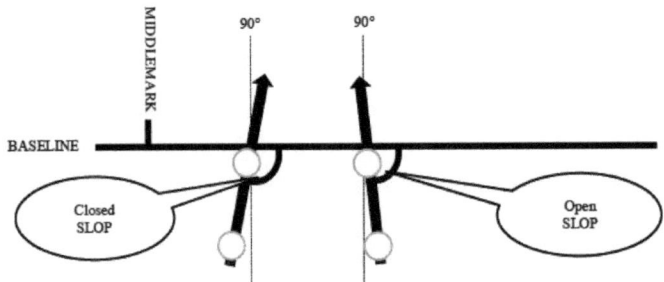

(SLOP), defined as „closed" (>90° to the baseline) or „open" (<90° to the baseline)

Markers on acromion, right and left = ◯

6

Figure 3

Lab documentation

Body marker positions

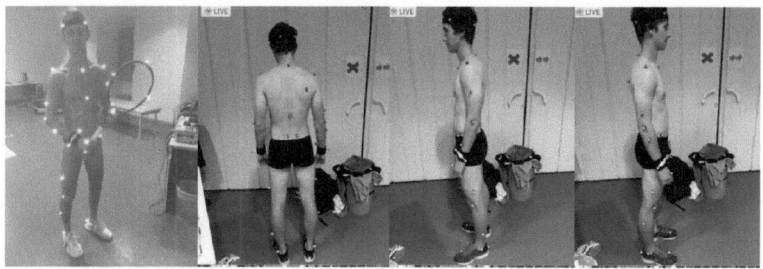

Figure 4

Lab documentation

Aligned position

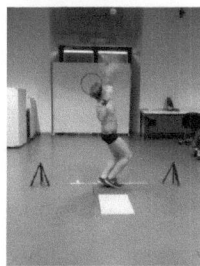

Figure 5

Lab documentation

Not aligned position

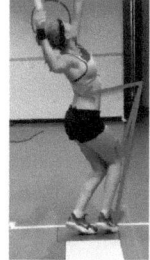

Kinetic values

SLOP is defined as the toss movement directly before the hitting hand and the racket head cock downwards (Figures 2a). At this point, the athlete chooses to position his shoulders in a particular preferred orientation line in relation to the baseline (see In Situ Capture: Figure 2a, 2b, 4 and 5). The SLOP instantly before ball impact is explained as; a. both feet are on the ground, b. the knees are bent, c. the hitting elbow points backwards, and d. the tossing non-serving arm aims (with arm extended) the ball at the highest point (after toss, Figure 2a). The SLOP of the serve was chosen as a measurement value, because no external influences impact the consistency or reproducibility of the position. Therefore, the Vicon SLOP test is considered to be reliable and reproducible (see Statistical methods).

Statistical methods

The analyses were calculated using SPSS (version 1.0.0.1213). Mean and SD values for the serve trials were computed for 31 recorded players during SLOP (Table 3). As a reproducibility value, the mean of five recorded trials per player in the statistics (see In Situ Capture) was used. The chi-squared goodness of fit test based on a one-sample test was used. The expected values were calculated to 50%. Level of significance was established at $p<0.05$. To investigate the hypothesis chi-squared calculation with one-sample test was used. The observed values were compared with the expected values. The expected value of SII/A1 was set to 35% crossed ED and 65% consistent ED (general opinion on ED, see study I). The expected value of SII/A2 is based on the results of the SII/A1 results (45% crossed ED and 55% consistent ED). Level of significance was established at $p<0.05$.

Figure 6

Study overview - research chart observed values

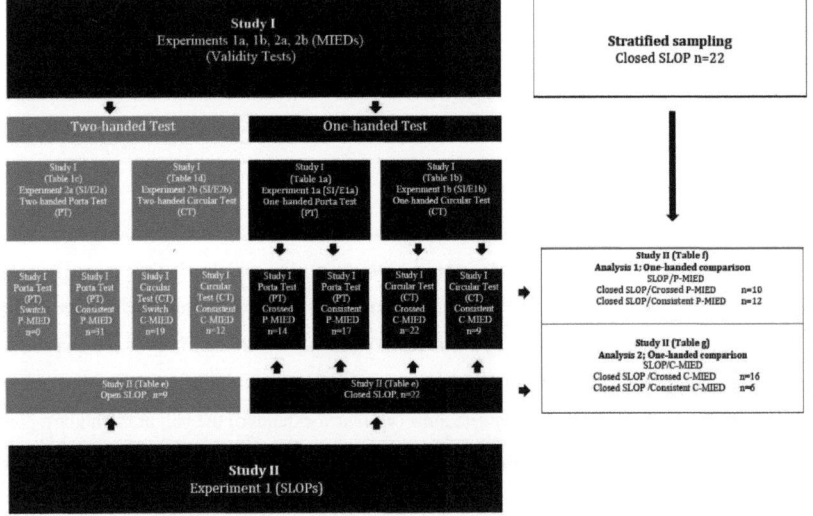

8

Results

The chi-squared results (Table 1 and Table 3) demonstrate that 22 (71%) of the 31 players preferred a closed SLOP, whereas nine (29%) of the 31 players preferred an open SLOP, $p=0.02$. To the best of our knowledge there are no studies to compare with. Therefore, the expected value of E1 was set to 50%. The experiment demonstrates that more players chose a closed SLOP instead of an open SLOP. Therefore, the closed SLOP/P-MIED (A1) result was compared with closed SLOP/C-MIED (A2) results in the analysis.

Analysis 1 - A1; comparison of closed SLOP with one-handed crossed and consistent P-MIED

The analysis A1 (Table 2a) focused on the closed SLOP in comparison to crossed respectively consistent P-MIED. The chi-squared result revealed that 10 (45%) players out of the 22 closed SLOP group showed a combination of closed SLOP and crossed eye dominance (P-MIED/) and 12 (55%) out of the 22 players showed a consistent P-MIED. The expected value was set to crossed $n=8$ (35%) and consistent $n=14$ (65%) in accordance to the general opinion about ED.

Analysis 2 - A2; comparison of the P-MIED with C-MIED

The final analysis (A2) compared the results of the closed SLOP/crossed P-MIED with closed SLOP/crossed C-MIED and closed SLOP/consistent P-MIED with closed SLOP/consistent C-MIED. The result of the A1 (P-MIEDs) was used as the expected value for A2. The A1 revealed that 10 out of the 22 closed SLOPs showed a crossed P-MIED result (Table 2a). A2 showed that 16 (73%) out of the 22 players with a closed SLOP showed a crossed C-MIED, whereas six (27%) players with a closed SLOP showed a consistent C-MIED ($n=6$) (Table 2b). Thus, the comparison of the results of P-MIED and C-MIED demonstrate that 6 players (50%) out of 12 players with a closed SLOP/consistent PT result changed their ED from consistent to crossed when they performed the one-handed CT. This is significant difference ($p=0.01$; Table 2b) and shows that manual motor tasks may have an effect on the ED and consequently be important for an optimized SLOP.

9

Table 1, 2a and 2b

Results of chi-squared tests of Study I (Experiments 1a, 1b, 2a and 2b) and Study II (Experiment 1 and analyses 1 and 2) observed and expected values, their proportions and distribution.

X^2 (df1, n=31) = 5.452			
Experiment	**Observed value**	**Expected value**	**p-value** $p= 0.02$
[1]CS	n=22 (71%)	n=15.5 (50%)	
[2]OS	n=9 (29%)	n=15.5 (50%)	

Table 1

Study II / Experiment 1; One-sample test - Goodness of Fit

Closed and Open SLOP [1]CS: Closed SLOP; [2]OS: Open SLOP

X^2 (df1, n=22) = 0.786				
Experiment	**Observed value**	**Expected value**	**p-value** $p=0.37$	**Table 2a** *Study II* */Analysis*
[3]CSCr1PM	10* (45%)	8 (35%)		
[4]CSCn1PM	12* (55%)	14 (65%)		

1 Only closed SLOP with one-handed crossed or consistent P-MIED

[3]CSCr1PM: Closed SLOP/Crossed P-MIED; [4]CSCn1PM: Closed SLOP/Consistent

C-MIED

X^2 (df1, n=22) = 6.6			
Experiment	**Observed value**	**Expected value** CSCr1PM; OV*	**p-value** $p=0.01$
[5]CSCr1CM	16 (73%)	10 (45%)*	
[6]CSCn1CM	6 (27%)	12 (55%)*	

Table 2b

Study II / Analysis 2

SLOP/C-MIED Comparison Only one-handed crossed with closed or open

[5]CSCr1CM: Closed SLOP/Crossed C-MIED; [6]CSCn1CM: Closed SLOP/Consistent

C-MIED

10

Discussion

The aim of the study was to investigate the association of previous presented MIEDs (Study I; Dahlbo et al., 2020) with the shoulder loading position (SLOP) in the tennis serve. The most important findings of the current study (Study II) were; first, that the personal SLOP in the tennis serve was documented and showed a significant higher frequency of closed SLOPs than the open SLOP; then, that closed SLOP combined with the one-handed P-MIED showed significant different results than did closed SLOP combined with one-handed C-MIED. These are important findings, because it shows that screening of MIEDs and SLOPs may contribute to our understanding of a player's personal choice of serving technique in tennis. To our knowledge, this study is the first to show that the manual motor system may contribute to a player's MIED classification, which, in turn, permits C-MIED and SLOP results to be evaluated for serve assessment in tennis. The results does not reveal why crossed C-MIED players seem to be more common in a closed SLOP than in the consistent group of the study sample. Nevertheless, since this is the first study to describe and evaluate C-MIED in comparison with P-MIED and SLOP assessment, no other studies are available for the purpose of comparison. With regard to practical implications, some examples below clarify the possible advantages and disadvantages for players who show a consistent versus a crossed respectively crossed-consistent, ipsilateral-consistent and crossed-switched C-MIED. Previous experiments (Dahlbo et al., 2020) show that the right-handed players are using the same eye in both circle finger tests T1 and T2 (crossed-consistent; right-hand/left eye, left hand/left eye, ipsilateral-consistent; right-hand/right eye, left hand/right eye). Thus, it may be argued that crossed-consistent right-handers prefer a more closed SLOP, whereas ipsilateral-consistent right-handers may favor an open SLOP. It can be argued that crossed-switch (two-handed; right-hand/left eye, left hand/right eye) C-MIED tennis players may use both eyes and hands interchangeably as required in order to themselves solve and optimize immediate motor challenges. Crossed-consistent C-MIED players might have abilities that are similar to those of ipsilateral-consistent players. However, they may differ in the SLOP. A crossed-consistent C-MIED player and an ipsilateral-consistent C-MIED player use the same eye regardless of which hand they are using. However, both crossed-consistent and ipsilateral-consistent C-MIEDs can be more consistent when assuming the

11

loading position (fewer choices and thus less need for adjustment) than can crossed-switch players.

The fact that players with a crossed (right hand/left eye) C-MIED are more frequent in the closed group, but are found in both the closed and the open SLOP sample group can be explained as an effect of the hand/finger activation sequence at the beginning of a swing (Figure 1). It may be argued that, in this case, right-handed players unconsciously choose a hand activation sequence (instinctively or as taught to them) and thus activate a preferred eye, which might favor certain SLOP. Hence, crossed-switch C-MIED tennis players might allow the left eye to take command by activating the right hand first (firm grip) and vice versa. The left-consistent player always activates the left eye and the right-consistent player always activates the right eye, regardless of which hand is being used. Ipsilateral consistent C-MIED (right hand/right-eyed players and vice versa for left-handers) and crossed-consistent C-MIED players (T2) might not easily adjust to a position that is not ideal for them and may need optimized and clear instructions, thus suggesting that they might be forced to stay in the learned SLOP. A centrally placed toss (frontal in relation to the body and placed frontal between the legs, player sideways to the net) may be more beneficial for a ipsilateral-consistent player (RH/RE-LH/RE), so the shoulder does not turn forward too early as a result of the personal C-MIED. A toss sideways towards the net in a sideways position might be very difficult for a right-handed ipsilateral-consistent C-MIED player, whereas a toss by a crossed-switch C-MIED player may be more flexible thanks to the ability to adapt and instantly interchange the sequence between both hands and eyes. Left-consistent C-MIED players can also toss the ball forwards towards the net and might show a consistent movement once it is properly learned. Moreover, the crossed-switch C-MIED player might show a greater ability to hit the ball on the way up or play serve and volley where the ability to toss the ball forwards (towards the net) is important and the hands and eyes need to interlink rapidly.

The presented results provide new insights into the relationship between hand-eye coordination and SLOP, with specific focus on the one-handed C-MIED. The results appear to be important for the assessment of skill development in tennis serve and contribute to a clearer understanding of visuomotor coaching. However, further studies are needed to strengthen, extend and diversify the presented hypotheses. Consequently, instructions aimed at having a student copy a successful top player, who might have a completely different C-MIED than the student, might indeed be counterproductive and should be reconsidered. However, it is important to understand that a consistent C-MIED might be at least as beneficial long-term once an appropriate technique has been learned. Moreover, it deserves to be mentioned that the study's results do not say anything about a player's success. This remains to be examined in future studies.

Strengths and limitations

The various nationalities of the studied players with different backgrounds increase the generalizability of the results (see Methods), and the functional design of the study has a strong link to the practical testing procedure that can be used on an everyday basis. New hypotheses may be derived from the presented results and may be useful and adaptable for further studies concerning tennis serving technique. The Vicon Test can be considered 100% reliable, which strengthens the validity of our recordings. The investigators' specific tennis experience is another strength because of the challenge to decide exact SLOP and the potential risk of misclassification. Some limitations of this study should be addressed. Tennis is a three-dimensional sport and involves many different strokes. Therefore, extracting one single stroke and one position of that stroke (SLOP) may be a limitation. Recordings with the eight-camera Vicon system may be a limitation due to the fast and complex three-dimensional motion in the tennis serve. Therefore, more cameras might be beneficial to capture more specific details (markers) during the fast serve motion. Finally, the study did not evaluate the quality (rhythm, coordination, equilibrium, balance, power, accuracy) of the serve, which may be a limitation to fully analyzing the success (ranking, tournament victories) of a player's serving ability.

Future perspective

Future research on a larger scale should involve more tennis players from different countries. Left-handers should also be examined.

Vicon recordings

More Vicon cameras should be involved for excellent and totally flawless biomechanical high-speed three-dimensional recordings. Evaluations using electroencephalography (EEG) when executing the HED test with the finger muscles and during active serving as well as electromyography *(EMG)* during assumption of the loading position are suggested for additional studies. Fingertip grip sensors can be applied to determine which hand a player primarily uses (the first activity, right or left hand) when delivering a serve. Finally, we recommend that the results showing the quality of the serve (placement and power) be additionally evaluated in future studies. The complexity of three-dimensional tennis biomechanics and MIED requires further research to investigate the challenging mechanisms behind this C-MIED/SLOP phenomenon. Therefore, this study should be considered a gate-opener and should support future studies of C-MIED and SLOP screening results and their role in the assessment of the tennis serve.

Practical applications

In view of the presented results the benefits and possibilities of the C-MIED and SLOP screening procedure (see C-MIED procedure) for assessment of the tennis serve may be presented in coach training programs to raise the sensibility and awareness of hand-eye dominance in coaching. Furthermore, inclusion of the HED procedure (see below) in daily skill training should be considered with the aim to avoid unnecessary basic technical errors and mandatory assessment routine.

The study suggests that the C-MIED procedure be taken into consideration when:

a. the coach notices an asymmetric (rhythm, coordination) movement during the serve process.
b. the coach notices that the player cannot follow technical instructions
c. the player lacks power in his serve.
d. the coach observes unnecessary movements within the preparation process like „dancing" (back and forth or up and down), knee or elbow and wrist deviations (waiter's serve).

e. the coach cannot decide if the player is using „non-fit" taught movements or if a deviation/adjustment occurs because of an unintentional „non-fit" sequence action of the hand.

The evaluation process works step by step. For optimal assessment of a tennis serve, we recommend that the process be administered in exactly the form suggested below.

C-MIED procedure:

1. First, explore the player's closed or open SLOP ($\geq$90° or <90° in relation to the baseline; see Introduction and Methods).

2. Then, perform the CT to assess the athlete's hand-eye dominance.

3. Next, match the one-handed crossed CT result and the closed versus the open SLOP (because crossed C-MIED appears to be more common in the study sample).

4. Finally, if no explanations are found, extend the test process and match right hand/right eye C-MIED (consistent C-MIED) versus closed and open SLOP.

5. The CT test is intended only as a screening tool and should not be used as a diagnosis instrument. That means that the results do not confirm a clear serve diagnosis plan, but identify the player's personal hand-eye dominance. Therefore, the CT procedure should be only one part of an extensive evaluation process including various other methods.

The CT process tool used as a basic fundament to develop an observational tool to evaluate the individual hand-eye coordination preference. The study suggest that the CT-tool might facilitate the evaluation in tennis serve mechanics without expensive equipment. There are several advantages to this type of analysis. First, it is mobile to practice or tournament sites and can be implemented on court. Thus, coaches and health care professionals must be able to easily identify mechanical flaws within the service motion to improve performance and diminish possible injury risk. However, there is no direct correlation between the findings of this analysis and either the incidence of injuries or the prevention of injuries or performance. Future studies need to investigate this procedure as one of the primary outcomes in both serve performance and injury related studies.

The study investigated the reliability of a field-based tool by using a personal hand-

15

eye prefence (C-MIED) and a prefered SLOP used to grade the preferences of the tennis serve. It was hypothesized that it is possible to find a manual influence of the eye dominance and its association of SLOP in tennis serve. The thesis describes a statistically significant association between the crossed C-MIED and the SLOP in the tennis serve.

Conclusions

The study describes an association between a C-MIED and the SLOP in the tennis serve. The findings showed a good reliability and validity and may have an impact on skill training and serving technique in tennis.

Acknowledgments

The authors express their gratitude to Prof. Dr Peter Federolf and Dr Thomas Haid at the Department for Sport Science, University of Innsbruck, Austria, for the 2nd supervision of the study and for permitting us to use the required facilities and Univ.-Prof. Dr Martin Krismer at the Medical University of Innsbruck for the 1st supervision of the study. The authors also feel it is important to express their gratitude to the players, parents and coaches of the Alexander Raschke Tennis Academy in Munich, Germany, and the Estess Academy in Tyrol, Austria, who intensely supported the project.

Table 3

Shoulder position in relation to the baseline - CT

			EVALUATION SHEET – STUDY 2		
Respondent (R)	**Gender**	**Allocation –**	**Circular Manual Motor**	**Angle to the Baseline**	
	M: Male F: Female	**Serve Groups**	**Task**	**☐ = Shoulder (Acromion)**	
R01-31	**M or F**	**OS: open stance**	**Experiment I**	**☐ mean**	**SD**
		CS: closed stance	**One-handed CT**		
01. R20-S25	M	CS	RH/LE Right Hand/Left Eye	105.6798032	3.650626825
02. R27-S32	M	CS	RH/LE Right Hand/Left Eye	90.10794352	2.341765188
03. R31-S36	M	CS	RH/LE Right Hand/Left Eye	93.6282671	2.366097709
04. R11-S11	F	CS	RH/LE Right Hand/Left Eye	103.5324056	2.316989986
05. R01-S01	M	CS	RH/LE Right Hand/Left Eye	100.5756812	2.718215469
06. R07-S07	M	CS	RH/LE Right Hand/Left Eye	110.219207	2.486159832
07. R19-S23	M	CS	RH/LE Right Hand/Left Eye	95.6765251	1.538219069
08. R21-S26	M	CS	RH/LE Right Hand/Left Eye	108.5235191	1.994725376
09. R28-S33	M	CS	RH/LE Right Hand/Left Eye	109.152397	4.105383497
10. R36-S41	M	CS	RH/LE Right Hand/Left Eye	105.6539684	1.366297348
11. R10-S10	F	CS	RH/LE Right Hand/Left Eye	115.5441361	3.046914438
12. R17-S21	F	CS	RH/LE Right Hand/Left Eye	96.59619219	7.059088083
13. R25-S30	F	CS	RH/LE Right Hand/Left Eye	91.04803508	3.322942877
14. R05-S05	M	CS	RH/LE Right Hand/Left Eye	95.61987469	2.291745519
15. R24-S29	M	CS	RH/LE Right Hand/Left Eye	99.95086939	0.991288398
16. R34-S39	M	CS	RH/LE Right Hand/Left Eye	108.5128737	2.256284171
17. R16-S18	F	CS	RH/RE Right Hand/Right Eye	96.21849794	2.23217042
18. R33-S38	F	CS	RH/RE Right Hand/Right Eye	110.8323104	1.672612708
19. R02-S02	M	CS	RH/RE Right Hand/Right Eye	103.4627534	5.741665973
20. R14-S16	M	CS	RH/RE Right Hand/Right Eye	120.7882217	1.18837275
21. R29-S34	M	CS	RH/RE Right Hand/Right Eye	96.85489601	3.028628548
22. R30-S35	M	CS	RH/RE Right Hand/Right Eye	90.15651576	15.10434002
23. R04-S04	F	OS	RH/LE Right Hand/Left Eye	82.31441678	3.52251124
24. R32-S37	F	OS	RH/LE Right Hand/Left Eye	70.59115929	2.437519085
25. R15-S17	M	OS	RH/LE Right Hand/Left Eye	76.21557582	2.457527411
26. R26-S31	M	OS	RH/LE Right Hand/Left Eye	84.45164011	3.218566674
27. R09-S09	F	OS	RH/LE Right Hand/Left Eye	87.46129886	5.925572166
28. R12-S12	M	OS	RH/LE Right Hand/Left Eye	87.97574562	1.577094682
29. R13-S14	M	OS	RH/RE Right Hand/Right Eye	78.35609573	3.15534838
30. R18-S22	M	OS	RH/RE Right Hand/Right Eye	66.82099784	2.48702193
31. R22-S27	M	OS	RH/RE Right Hand/Right Eye	79.54734078	1.977732468

Table 4

Shoulder position in relation to the baseline - PT

<table>
<tr><th colspan="6">EVALUATION SHEET – STUDY 2</th></tr>
<tr>
<th>Respondent (R)</th>
<th>Gender
M: Male F: Female</th>
<th>Allocation –
Serve Groups</th>
<th>Circular Manual
Motor Task</th>
<th colspan="2">Angle to the Baseline
◻ = Shoulder (Acromion)</th>
</tr>
<tr>
<th>R01-31</th>
<th>M or F</th>
<th>OS: open stance
CS: closed stance</th>
<th>One-handed PT</th>
<th>◻ mean</th>
<th>SD</th>
</tr>
<tr><td>01. R20-S25</td><td>M</td><td>CS</td><td>RH/LE
Right Hand/Left Eye</td><td>105.6798032</td><td>3.650626825</td></tr>
<tr><td>02. R27-S32</td><td>M</td><td>CS</td><td>RH/LE
Right Hand/Left Eye</td><td>90.10794352</td><td>2.341765188</td></tr>
<tr><td>03. R31-S36</td><td>M</td><td>CS</td><td>RH/LE
Right Hand/Left Eye</td><td>93.6282671</td><td>2.366097709</td></tr>
<tr><td>04. R11-S11</td><td>F</td><td>CS</td><td>RH/LE
Right Hand/Left Eye</td><td>103.5324056</td><td>2.316989986</td></tr>
<tr><td>05. R01-S01</td><td>M</td><td>CS</td><td>RH/LE
Right Hand/Left Eye</td><td>100.5756812</td><td>2.718215469</td></tr>
<tr><td>06. R07-S07</td><td>M</td><td>CS</td><td>RH/LE
Right Hand/Left Eye</td><td>110.219207</td><td>2.486159832</td></tr>
<tr><td>07. R19-S23</td><td>M</td><td>CS</td><td>RH/LE
Right Hand/Left Eye</td><td>95.6765251</td><td>1.538219069</td></tr>
<tr><td>08. R21-S26</td><td>M</td><td>CS</td><td>RH/LE
Right Hand/Left Eye</td><td>108.5235191</td><td>1.994725376</td></tr>
<tr><td>09. R28-S33</td><td>M</td><td>CS</td><td>RH/LE
Right Hand/Left Eye</td><td>109.152397</td><td>4.105383497</td></tr>
<tr><td>10. R36-S41</td><td>M</td><td>CS</td><td>RH/LE
Right Hand/Left Eye</td><td>105.6539684</td><td>1.366297348</td></tr>
<tr><td>11. R10-S10</td><td>F</td><td>CS</td><td>RH/RE
Right Hand/Right Eye</td><td>115.5441361</td><td>3.046914438</td></tr>
<tr><td>12. R17-S21</td><td>F</td><td>CS</td><td>RH/RE
Right Hand/Right Eye</td><td>96.59619219</td><td>7.059988083</td></tr>
<tr><td>13. R25-S30</td><td>F</td><td>CS</td><td>RH/RE
Right Hand/Right Eye</td><td>91.04803508</td><td>3.322942877</td></tr>
<tr><td>14. R05-S05</td><td>M</td><td>CS</td><td>RH/RE
Right Hand/Right Eye</td><td>95.61987469</td><td>2.291745519</td></tr>
<tr><td>15. R24-S29</td><td>M</td><td>CS</td><td>RH/RE
Right Hand/Right Eye</td><td>99.95086939</td><td>0.991288398</td></tr>
<tr><td>16. R34-S39</td><td>M</td><td>CS</td><td>RH/RE
Right Hand/Right Eye</td><td>108.5128737</td><td>2.256284171</td></tr>
<tr><td>17. R16-S18</td><td>F</td><td>CS</td><td>RH/RE
Right Hand/Right Eye</td><td>96.21849794</td><td>2.23217042</td></tr>
<tr><td>18. R33-S38</td><td>F</td><td>CS</td><td>RH/RE
Right Hand/Right Eye</td><td>110.8323104</td><td>1.672612708</td></tr>
<tr><td>19. R02-S02</td><td>M</td><td>CS</td><td>RH/RE
Right Hand/Right Eye</td><td>103.4627534</td><td>5.741665973</td></tr>
<tr><td>20. R14-S16</td><td>M</td><td>CS</td><td>RH/RE
Right Hand/Right Eye</td><td>120.7882217</td><td>1.18837275</td></tr>
<tr><td>21. R29-S34</td><td>M</td><td>CS</td><td>RH/RE
Right Hand/Right Eye</td><td>96.85489601</td><td>3.028628548</td></tr>
<tr><td>22. R30-S35</td><td>M</td><td>CS</td><td>RH/RE
Right Hand/Right Eye</td><td>90.15651576</td><td>15.10434002</td></tr>
<tr><td>23. R04-S04</td><td>F</td><td>OS</td><td>RH/LE
Right Hand/Left Eye</td><td>82.31441678</td><td>3.52251124</td></tr>
<tr><td>24. R32-S37</td><td>F</td><td>OS</td><td>RH/LE
Right Hand/Left Eye</td><td>70.59115929</td><td>2.437519085</td></tr>
<tr><td>25. R15-S17</td><td>M</td><td>OS</td><td>RH/LE
Right Hand/Left Eye</td><td>76.21557582</td><td>2.457527411</td></tr>
<tr><td>26. R26-S31</td><td>M</td><td>OS</td><td>RH/LE
Right Hand/Left Eye</td><td>84.45164011</td><td>3.218566674</td></tr>
<tr><td>27. R09-S09</td><td>F</td><td>OS</td><td>RH/RE
Right Hand/Right Eye</td><td>87.46129886</td><td>5.925572166</td></tr>
<tr><td>28. R12-S12</td><td>M</td><td>OS</td><td>RH/RE
Right Hand/Right Eye</td><td>87.97574562</td><td>1.577094682</td></tr>
<tr><td>29. R13-S14</td><td>M</td><td>OS</td><td>RH/RE
Right Hand/Right Eye</td><td>78.35609573</td><td>3.15534838</td></tr>
<tr><td>30. R18-S22</td><td>M</td><td>OS</td><td>RH/RE
Right Hand/Right Eye</td><td>66.82099784</td><td>2.48702193</td></tr>
<tr><td>31. R22-S27</td><td>M</td><td>OS</td><td>RH/RE
Right Hand/Right Eye</td><td>79.54734078</td><td>1.977732468</td></tr>
</table>

Reference List

Campbell, A., O'Sullivan, P., Straker, L., Elliott, B., & Reid, M. (2013). Back Pain in Tennis Players: A Link with Lumbar Serve Kinematics and Range of Motion. *Medicine and Science in Sports and Exercise*, 46(2), 351-357.

Dahlbo, H., Flatz, M., Federolf, P., & Krismer, M. (2020). Eye dominance testing: An exploration of the conventional standard eye dominance Porta Test in comparison with a circular manually influenced eye dominance Test. *Department for Sport Science, University of Innsbruck, Austria, Non-published.*

Elliott, B., & Wood, G. (1983). The biomechanics of the foot-up and foot-back tennis service techniques. *The Australian Journal of Sports Sciences,* 3(2), 3-6.

Elliott, B., Marshall, R., & Noffal, G. (1995). Contributions of upper limb segment rotations during the power serve in tennis. *Journal of Applied Biomechanics*, 11, 433-442.

Elliott, B., Fleisig, G., Nicholls, R., & Escamilia R. (2003). Technique effects on upper limb loading in the tennis serve. *Journal of Science and Medicine in Sport / Sports Medicine Australia,* 6(1), 76-87.

Ford, K., & Myer, G., & Hewett, T. (2007). Reliability of Landing 3D Motion Analysis. Medicine and science in sports and exercise. 39. 2021-8. 10.1249/mss.0b013e318149332d.

Girard, O., Micallef, J., & Millet, G. (2005). Lower-limb activity during the power serve intennis: effects of performance level. *Medicine and Science in Sports and Exercise,* 37(6), 1021-1029.

Girard, O., Micallef, J., & Millet, G. (2007). Influence of restricted knee motion during the flat first serve in tennis. *Journal of Strength and Conditioning research,* 21(3), 950-957.

Khan, A., & Crawford, J. (2001). Ocular dominance reverses as a function of horizontal gaze angle. *Vision Research,* 41, 1743–1748.

Kibler, W. (1995). Biomechanical analysis of the shoulder during tennis activities. *Clinical Sports Medicine,* 14, 79-85.

Kovacs, M., & Ellenbecker, T. (2011). An 8-stage model for evaluating the tennis serve, implications for performance enhancement and injury prevention. *Sports Health,* 3(6), 504–513.

Martin C., Kulpa R., Ropars M., Delamarche P., & Bideau B. (2013). Identification of temporal pathomechanical factors during the tennis serve. *Medical Science of Sports Exercise*, 45(11), 2113-2119.

Martin, C., Bideau, B., Bideau, N., Nicolas, G., Delamarche, P., & Kulpa, R. (2014). Energy flow analysis during the tennis serve: Comparison between injured and noninjured tennis players. *American Journal of Sports Medicine*, 42(11), 2751–2760.

Martin C., Bideau B., Ropars M., Delamarche P., & Kulpa R. (2014). Upper limb joint kinetic analysis during tennis serve: Assessment of competitive level on efficiency and injury risks. *Scandinavian Journal of Medical Science in Sports*, 24(4), 700-707.

Toyoshima, S., Hoshikawa, T., & Miyashita, M. (1974). Contributions of body parts to throwing performance. *Biomechanics IV*. Baltimore: University Park Press;169-174.

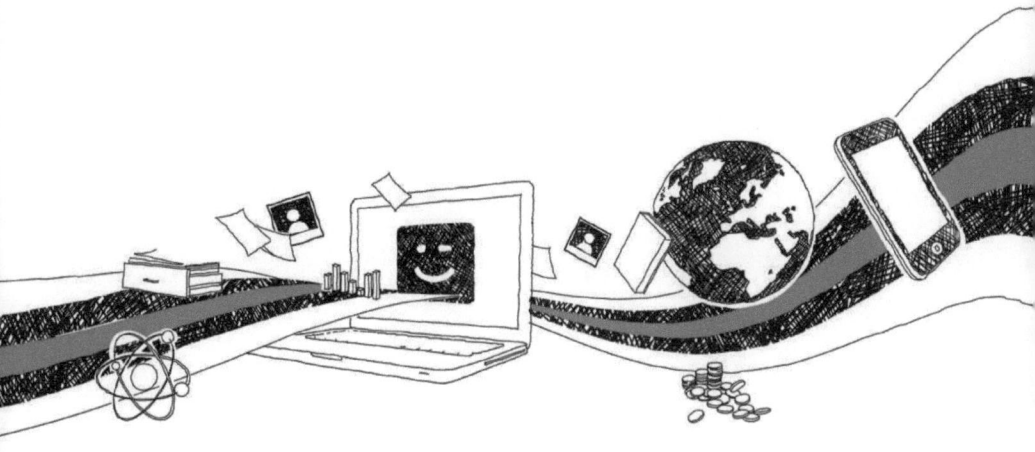
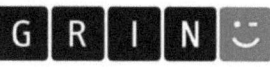